ME
AND
MY HABITS

Tips on how to develop good habits and get over bad habits in simple ways.

Copyright©2021 Carly Jones

All Rights Reserved

TABLE OF CONTENT

Table of Contents

INTRODUCTION

Our habits consciously and unconsciously have led to many being very wealthy and many being poor.

Our habits have led to the success of many relationships and also failure of many relationships.

Our habits have led to the success of many students and likewise the failure of many students.

Whatever our level today, our habits have contributed greatly to it.

When we realize that our habits have a lot to do with either our success or failure in the present and future, then we ought to pay attention to the habits we are forming today.

Good habits may not be easy to build but when we think of the gains that comes from it, then it is worth building that good habits.

Bad habits may not be easy to let go, but when we realize the cost of failure, then it is worth doing everything within our power to overcome the bad habits.

The book - Me and My Habits, is the book for all who want to excel greatly.

CHAPTER ONE

What is a habit? A habit is a behavior that is repeated routinely. This behavior can be an activity, a daily practice, or a way of life.

A habit is also a standard of behavior that can be created through regular reiteration.

Basically, a habit is something that you do frequently or consistently, without considering everything.

Shaping a Habit

While framing a habit, we need to recognize three things:

1.   Generate

2.   Repetitive

3.   Result

Generate

What could it be that generate the habit? This can be, for example, a morning awaken style, which is enacted by your morning timer. After hearing the morning timer ringing, you are set off to awaken from your bed at that point continue into a set daily schedule.

Every one of the habits will have some type of trigger, regardless of whether the trigger is clear actual signals, or more subtle mental prompts. What's more, you may have to think all the more profoundly to distinguish a more subtle trigger.

Trigger exist as far as possible and start a habit. This is the idea of a habit.

Accordingly, when you start to shape a habit, you ought to get mindful of the trigger. It will assist you with properly starting a habit, as you need to.

<u>Repetitive</u>

A routine is the foundation of a habit. This is the repetition of a social activity. You will repeat the behavior activity in a habit.

In the event that you are deliberately framing a habit, you will need to invest your energy thinking cautiously what the behavior action(s) of your standard will be about. Settling on the behavior action(s) will likewise be controlled by the following significant thing of a habit – result.

Result

After you played out an everyday practice (your habit), there will be a result. You may anticipate that your outcome should be a standard assignment finished. This normal assignment can be pretty much as straightforward as the habit for brushing your teeth toward the beginning of the day.

The result is you having lovely white teeth from the habit.

The result from a habit can likewise be more mind boggling. A few results may be hard to screen and check. For instance, a more extensive habit for practicing good eating habits, which will be hard to screen and check. Envision, you generally eat organic products, as a component of the habit for practicing good eating habits, yet what amount improved wellbeing does the eaten natural products contribute?

A sound result will be hard to measure. You won't know whether sound is dictated by physical or potentially enthusiastic prosperity. This is an unpredictable result.

At the point when you intentionally structure a habit, consider cautiously the result your habit will accomplish. Keep your result as something quantifiable. Thus, it will be simpler to follow the exhibition of your new habit.

Depending on the situation, with the painstakingly thought result, you may have to change the daily schedule to line up with the target of your result.

Time Needed To Create a Habit

After you have built up a habit, you need to invest the energy to routinely follow it. When you invested energy over and again on the habit, it will end up being your natural. At times, you probably won't have to deliberately think about the habit you are performing. It will occur without your cognizant idea.

To accomplish a grounded habit in your life it will require roughly about a month of consistent repetition.

Be that as it may, the time taken for building another habit can vary incredibly. This relies upon the idea of the actual habit. In the event that your habit is basic and can be repeated rapidly inside a short time period, it may take more limited to set up the habit. Something else, if your habit is more convoluted and require an extensive length to do, it may take longer than a month.

Changing a Habit

Utilizing the above three aspects of creating a habit, you can devise an arrangement to change your habit. On the off chance that you are hoping to change your habit, you should consider the - generate, repetitive and result of the habit. Wonder why you need to change the habit, is it for another result? Or on the other hand, is the current result not being accomplished by the daily practice? You need to trigger the habit in some other manner? With your responses to the above questions, you will actually want to recognize obviously the phase of habit you need to change. Knowing the stage that require changes will let you successfully plan a change.

In the event that it is another outcome you look for, you should choose what new outcome the habit needs to accomplish. At that point, you will probably have to make changes in accordance with the daily practice also.

On the off chance that it is a standard change to more readily arrive at the current result, you should initially assess why the current routine isn't working. In light of your assessment, you should settle on the suitable changes to your present daily practice.

For certain great habits, you may be considering accomplishing a greater amount of it. This can be effectively added by new triggers. The expansion of triggers will assist with provoking your everyday practice. Consequently, you will accomplish a greater amount of the habit.

On the off chance that you are hoping to dispose of a negative behavior pattern, the least demanding will be to focus on the trigger piece of a habit. For this situation, you could essentially try not to be in a climate or circumstance that may trigger your habit.

Effectively, you can maintain a strategic distance from the habit.

Critically, while changing or eliminating a habit, it will take cognizant exertion and time. You should show restraint. Effectively recollect the change to your habit, and to do the habit when set off. Similarly, in the event that you are eliminating a habit, make sure to effectively maintain a strategic distance from the habit's trigger. This can be staying away from a climate or finding yourself mixed up with explicit circumstances.

CHAPTER TWO

Essential habits an individual should have

1. Start Your Day with Reflection

Various stressors may trigger as you go as the day progressed; reflection assists you with trying to avoid panicking prior to taking on the difficulties.

Reflection is a decent habit to have in the event that you need to be associated with what's huge in your life.

2. Be Thankful for What You Have

It's normal to sit around thinking about what's insufficient. You become drenched in those overwhelming difficulties. Nonetheless, challenges legitimize the presence of expectation. The lone methodology you need to quit zeroing in on your issues is to zero in on what you have.

Appreciation is a tried and true pathway to progress, wellbeing, and bliss. It diverts your concentration to what you have from what you need. Have a go at composing a rundown of things you're thankful for every day.

3. Smile

A real smile is a decent habit to have on the off chance that you need to discover profound, passionate, and mental genuine feelings of peace.

Smiling actuates the arrival of atoms that work towards battling pressure. The physiological condition of your body decides the condition of your brain. At the point when you frown, your brain takes signals identifying with sadness and hopelessness. Notwithstanding, when you change yourself by putting on a smile, you start to feel another degree of enthusiasm and liveliness.

At the point when you smile, you set a tone for carrying on with a more joyful life.

4. Start Your Day with a Sound Breakfast

Beginning your day with a sound breakfast is a decent habit to have and frames a vital piece of your life. By and by, a huge level of individuals avoid their morning meal every day.

On the off chance that you are tired hearing that morning meal is a critical part of your day, you are just battling reality. On the off chance that you need to turn out to be more fruitful, you need to have sound breakfast each day.

This habit isn't hard to shape in the event that you normally surge out the entryway each and every morning. You can get up prior to fix yourself a meal so you don't collapse during the day.

5. Figure out how to work out.

We need active work to remain solid. The advantages of normal exercise are very much reported. We need to discover practice schedules that are fun and match our individual tastes. Building up a decent exercise routine is a habit that will upsurge both the quantity and worth of your life.

One of the great habits to have is to practice your body and muscles consistently

6. Time Management

Another great habit is the demonstration of dealing with your time adequately. This goes far toward affecting your accomplishment.

Time management is which isolates the successful from the remainder of the world as we as a whole have a similar measure of time. How you influence time decides your capability to prevail throughout everyday life.

7. Set Day by day Objectives with Aims

Everybody has objectives, regardless of whether they identify with business or individual life. Actually, we're all tending towards a specific course. By and by, while long time objectives can offer you heading, it's your day by day objectives that assist you with creating term objectives that are fundamental for your prosperity.

Long time objectives may not give you the inspiration you need to keep on, however when you execute your transient achievements every day, you become started up, and you can defeat the difficulties that accompany taking on greater undertakings.

The fact of the matter is fruitful individuals don't set objectives without building up their aims.

8. Look for Motivation

It is typically hard to be propelled for an extensive period of time. Here and there, you become debilitate and want to abandon your objectives when things are not working out as expected.

A pragmatic way to deal with circumstances is to motivate yourself every day. At the point when you get up in the first part of the day (after reflection), observe some persuasive recordings, and let the account of extraordinary pioneers motivate you.

Motivation is the fuel for accomplishment since when you can consider it in your psyche, you can achieve it.

9. Save Consistently, Invest With All Carefulness

The vast majority neglect the meaning of putting something aside for the future when they are living in their current second.

Be that as it may, it isn't sufficient to save, and you should contribute your assets and be shrewd with them. On the off chance that you focus on this now, you will set yourself up for an existence of achievement later on. Guarantee you save in any event four months in your crisis account so you can be ready for any future crisis.

10. Financial plan and Track Your Spending

Planning is a decent habit to have, and it can affect your monetary life altogether. The cash you spend on excessive ways of life can be saved and put resources into your future all things being equal.

11. Grow great study habits.

Concentrating viably is an ability. Individuals that carry on with life to the fullest are long lasting students. They try constantly new things. One requirements to study and assemble new information in a compelling and productive way.

Figuring out how to consider and secure the information to succeed doesn't simply happen normally. It should be educated.

12. Never surrender!

It takes constancy in life to appreciate any sort of progress. Persistence is a habit. It is one that can be grown very much like some other. Try not to surrender amidst tough spot. You will get through.

13. Get on a decent timetable.

We need organization and routine in our lives. Our bodies anticipate it. They perform best when we work on a customary timetable. We particularly need to eat and rest about a similar time every day. As a parent, you should show your small kid this habit in his initial days. This standard stays with an individual their entire life and assists them with growing great work habits. Discover a timetable that works for you and stick to it!

14. Eat a healthy food.

Our cerebrums need the correct food to perform at their pinnacle. Try not to go to class or work on an empty stomach. Scholars need to prepare themselves right on time to eat a fair and solid eating routine. We will in general convey the habits we realize when we are youthful forward with us for a large portion of our lives. Figuring out how to eat right currently can maintain a strategic distance from numerous medical problems as it were.

15. Regard the climate.

We just have this one world and we rely upon it for our survival. Each individual have to do their part to protect what we have. Create habits that will assist you with being a decent ecological resident for a lifetime!

16. Struggle for greatness!

For what reason do a task in the event that you're not going to do it right? We need to build up the habit for giving each undertaking our best exertion. Greatness ought to be the standard we take a stab at taking all things together we do. We can't begin letting ourselves or our kids do the most un-conceivable to get by. In the event that we do, they will get not exactly the best outcomes from their work. Encouraging greatness presently will guarantee habits for progress will convey forward.

17. Live the Superb Guideline.

The Superb guideline is - we ought to figure out how to do to others what we need them to do to us. Think about the contention and misfortune that might have been stayed away from if individuals essentially applied the Superb Guideline taking all things together their connections. Assuming we make this a habit, we will discover significantly more accomplishment throughout everyday life. Regarding individuals, all things considered, and convictions is a sign of making every moment count.

18. Practice great cleanliness.

You truly can dress for progress! Habits like brushing your teeth two times every day and washing your hands consistently add to wellbeing, yet in addition lead to schedules that give one a more keen appearance. Initial feelings are incredible and are for the most part gotten from the manner in which an individual looks. Like it or not this is valid. Start today to guarantee you take the necessary steps to have an enduring decent effect.

19. Continuously come clean!

Reality regularly comes out if we need it to. Lying commonly confuses the circumstance and makes us look awful. It is vastly improved to simply build up the habit for coming clean in any event, when it is troublesome. This will save you a great deal of sorrow and hopelessness throughout everyday life.

20. Request what you need.

Build up the habit for requesting what you need. By what other method would you say you will get it? It is actually that basic. Regularly, when I ask, I'm astonished at how rapidly I get precisely what I needed. Simply check this one out. On the off chance that you are a parent, encourage your youngsters to ask others for what they need. This is genuinely a behavior you need to fall into place. It will fabricate certainty and confidence that will serve your children for eternity!

21. Be a consistent reader

Being a consistent reader is an expertise that regularly isolates the great students from those that battle. Turning into a consistent reader takes practice. The more you read and are perused to, the better you get. Reading has various advantages. It constructs one's jargon, grows the creative mind, and revives imagination. Make reading a daily practice!

22. Be prompt.

Showing up on time is essential to one's prosperity. Individuals consistently notice when you are late. It is a marker of whether you mean what you say and can be trusted. Try not to bring question about this into individuals' psyches by appearing later than anticipated. Make the habit for being reliable now and you will not need to stress.

23. Regard authority.

Inability to regard those in power positions can prompt a wide range of issues throughout everyday life. It doesn't make any difference whether it is your senior associate, a military official, or an instructor. Individuals in power have something important to take care of and regularly endeavored to get into the position they are in. They have the right to be treated with legitimate habits and respect.

24. Watch out for your otherworldly necessities.

We can't disregard our otherworldly necessities and really carry on with a full and compensating life. We should perceive that there is a higher force and seek after our confidence consistently. We may not exercise our convictions in the very same manner, yet I urge you to discover what works for you and investigate it to its profundities. A strong profound life will work well for you.

CHAPTER THREE

Essential habits of a good wife

1.   Study Your Better half

Become familiar with the things your husband likes or dislikes.

Indeed, even that little activity can help you begin shaping positive habits as a good wife.

I additionally know the interests my husband prefers, however I study the new things he discusses too.

You become a renewed individual like clockwork in view of the amount we develop and change through our encounters throughout everyday life. By considering your significant other and learning his preferences now, you will shape a positive habit to read your better half for quite a long time to come.

2.   Initiate Closeness

Marriage is a progressing demonstration of solidarity. Sex was made by God as a cozy second to occur between just a couple. Each opportunity you meet up as one, you are helped to remember the marriage agreement you made together and turn out to be more brought together as one.

It tends to be difficult for one individual to be the one in particular that starts seasons of closeness.

3.   Encourage Your Husband

We as a whole need consolation. There are such countless hard minutes in life where we feel like our endeavors are to no end. Discover approaches to support your husband that will explicitly lift him up in regions that you realize he feels feeble.

4.   Show Your Appreciation

Value your husband consistently, in any event, for things you consider nearly nothing, it goes far …

You don't lose anything from saying a straight-forward thank you every day.

5.   Learn the abilities of running a Home

Running a home takes a ton of work. From the financial plan to the clothing, to the cleaning and putting together, it appears there is continually something to do!

This is one of the habits for a decent wife since it will just form for quite a long time to come. In the event that you master abilities like sewing, cultivating, and cleaning now you can just improve at them! At that point when you have youngsters and a bigger obligation, your abilities will be adjusted and all set.

6.   Forgive

A decent wife need to figure out how to excuse her husband wrongs each and every day. Some of the time it tends to be very difficult to pardon, yet it is the thing that God calls us to do.

Without forgiveness, you will build walls, resentment, and deeper hurt.

On the off chance that you are thinking that it's hard to excuse your husband, it will be good to pray about it so God can help you in forgiving him.

7.   Engage in activities together.

Taking part in exercises together that you both appreciate is perhaps the most essential habit of a decent wife.

It should consistently be a priority.

8.   Treat Your Husband With Respect

It's one of the most practical habits of a good wife because as much as you need love from your husband, he needs respect from you. Begin assembling the establishment for a solid marriage today with deference!

9.   Submit To His Guidance

Obedience really shows your power as a lady. It demonstrates your capacity to be generous, experienced, and understanding. Conflicting with your physical longing isn't simple. At the point when a lady submit, she shows that she is sufficiently able to pick the proper thing.

10.   Ask His Assessment on All Choices

Work on asking your husband's assessment on everything. What's yours is his and what's his yours. Recall that you are brought together as one under Christ and in this way, you settle on choices together.

11.   Brag About Him

It will lift your better half up when you boast about him before others.

12.   Create A Serene Home

A decent wife ought to figure out how to make a tranquil home for her better half and kids.

CHAPTER FOUR

Essential habits of a good husband

1. Take a look at her

Take a look at your companion and let her realize that she's unique to you and you love her.

2. Be helpful

You should be a decent audience for your wife. Moreover, you need to offer her the appreciation she merits and the help she needs. Get into a routine of paying attention to your wife and not just simply hearing her.

3. Show physical and passionate warmth

You need to show her you love her through words and activities. Regardless of whether it's similarly just about as straightforward as clasping hands, or a startling embrace, spouses love it when husbands receive the habit for showing genuine fondness.

4. Praise her consistently

Your wife necessities praises as much as anybody, and they love it when spouses praise them frequently.

Praise her on her looks, or her abilities as a mother. It'll light up her day and reinforce your marriage. This is perhaps the most basic habits to execute.

5. Value and venerate her

You need to cherish your wife by loving her unreservedly. Let your priority be to make her happy and be willing to make sacrifices for her to be comfortable.

CHAPTER FIVE

Essential habits of a successful relationship

1. Continuously show regard to your partner

Showing respect to your partner is a habit that's worth having as it's a vital element for making an upbeat, solid and dependable relationship. At the point when you express regard towards your partner, you are communicating your adoration, acknowledgment, and warmth. At the point when you express discourtesy, you are communicating that you don't acknowledge your partner. Regarding your partner is tied in with esteeming them for who they are, including contrasts. You may have an alternate point of view yet this doesn't imply that you should affront your partner and put them down.

At the point when you experience conflicts, ensure that you regard your partner's disparities. This doesn't permit you to disregard your partner openly or before loved ones. Continuously show regard particularly when you have a conflict. There will be times where you disagree on an issue and it will be the means by which you handle this issue as a group that will have a significant effect.

2. Go strolling with your partner
Strolling with your partner advances great exercise and make happy chance to discuss various things.

It upgrades your relationship and brings you two together.

Choose with your partner how long and how regularly you might want to walk; the key factor is being in total agreement and ensuring that you settle on the psychological choice to set up this habit together.

3. Make cup of coffee for your partner in the morning

This humble gesture communicates love and regards to your partner. On the off chance that your partner likes to have cup of coffee in the morning, make this a habit and express love through this demonstration of administration. At the point when you carry some cup of coffee to your partner, it basically shows that you care and have your spouse in mind. This is a basic yet amazing habit for upbeat relationship.

4. Express optimistic features about your partner to other people

The habit for communicating positive features about your partner will help develop the association in your relationship. Despite what is generally expected, communicating negative ascribes about your partner will just form a tall divider among you. Do you know a couple that consistently contends openly and communicates negative characteristics about one another to companions? This is an unfortunate habit that in the long run obliterates a relationship. This negative example of behavior makes question, disengagement and absence of regard. Make a habit for communicating positive features to other people. This positive example of behavior makes esteem, affection and love.

5. Reconnect all through the day

We have such bustling timetables that interface with your partner for the duration of the day, that can make your partner to be less priority, however on the off chance that you need to have a cheerful, dependable relationship, reconnecting with your partner for the duration of the day is significant. It tends to be pretty much as straightforward as sending a caring book during your mid-day break or calling your partner.

6. Express appreciation to your partner consistently

Value your partner! It's pretty much as straightforward as that. Anyway you need to communicate appreciation in your relationship, do it. Do it each and every day. With regards to amazing habits for glad connections, it's tied in with communicating your appreciation to your partner. This can be leaving an adoration note prior to going to work or little blessing like bread roll, chocolate – whatever you realize that your partner likes.

7. Work all together towards objectives (short and long time)

A glad relationship centers on short and long time objectives. These objectives are both for every person and furthermore as a team. Miserable couples have nothing to anticipate throughout everyday life. They simply squander their energy on shallow hogwash and attempting to satisfy society's norm of bliss. Zero in inside your relationship on making, building up and achieving objectives.

Upbeat couples have objectives that are both little and large.

8. Cuddle in the mornings and nights

Set aside the effort to cuddle prior to beginning your day and prior to hitting the hay. This can be pretty much as straightforward as holding each other in bed for a couple of moments prior to beginning the day. Did you realize that actual touch delivers a chemical called Oxytocin? The more you experience actual touch with your partner, your oxytocin level increments. In the wake of a monotonous day of work, require significant investment prior to heading to sleep and nestle!

CHAPTER SIX

<u>10 Habits for Effective Pupils</u>

<u>1. Get Coordinated</u>. Making an arrangement for what you will do and when you will do it will ensure you're generally at the top - in a real sense.

<u>2. Set a timetable.</u> You need to check what works well for you – is it just after school or after you've had supper? Is it true that you are more beneficial in hour and a half squares or half-hour sprays? Discover a timetable that works for you, and stick to it.

<u>3. Rest</u>. Try not to think little of the significance of those eight hours of rest each night! Getting a decent night's rest will enhance your concentration and improve your working memory.

4. Pose inquiries. You're in school to learn, so don't be hesitant to do exactly that! Requesting help from an educator, a coach or your companions - is a certain method to ensure you genuinely comprehend the material.

5. Manage your learning space. Discover a spot that will expand your profitability. Regardless of whether it's your neighborhood library or simply the work area in your room, put to the side a learning space that you'll need to invest energy in.

6. Study. This one may be self-evident. Study rightly at all times as there are right and wrong way to study. Find out what works best for you, to study small portion of book daily or large portion at a time. Go over it regularly and avoid cramming.

7. Split it. Studying isn't enjoyable in any case, and driving yourself through a very long studying will make it worse. Split your studying into smaller bits and reward yourself when you finish each part will motivate you in achieving more.

8. Discover a learning group. Sitting down with a gathering of individuals who are learning very similar things as you is an incredible approach over confounding class material or get ready for a major test. You can test one another, reteach material, and ensure that everybody is in total agreement.

9. Take notes. Taking notes won't just keep you more active during class, however, it will likewise help you to focus on what you need to read when test time is around. It's a lot simpler to repeat your notes than to repeat your whole reading material!

10. Don't perform various tasks. Studies have shown that performing multiple tasks is truly incomprehensible.

CHAPTER SEVEN

Essential Productivity Habits

Follow these profitability habits in case you're not kidding about keeping focused towards whatever it is that you're endeavoring to accomplish throughout everyday life.

1. Follow a morning schedule.

Make an engaging morning schedule that you can use each and every morning to give you the greatest advantage in the day.

2. Make a day by day daily agenda.

Make an easy plan for the day each and every day with things to do that will draw you nearer and nearer to your objectives.

3. Recognize significant however not-pressing errands.

In time management, the significant however not pressing errands are those that will assist with moving you nearest to your drawn out objectives.

4. Track efficiency numbers every day.

Set aside the effort to follow everything. Down to the absolute last red penny, dollar, ounce, pound, gram or some other unit of measure. In the event that you do this, you can perceive examples to assist you with being gainful.

5. Do a week after week audit each day.

Go through what you accomplished toward the finish of each and every day and consider and stock of that so you can see your advancement.

<u>6. Disregard the immaterial.</u>

Disregard the things that are burning through your time yet that you will in general fixate on. While troublesome from the start, with training, this gets simpler.

<u>7. Take adequate breaks for the duration of the day.</u>

Little redirections from the job needing to be done can assist with intensifying efficiency.

<u>8. Picture the outcome.</u>

Perception is a colossal device in assisting you with surviving and mount the apparently impossible, assisting with being more profitable for the duration of the day.

9. Dodge interferences and interruptions.

Interferences and interruptions can break the progression of reasoning and it does requires a long time to get once more into the notch subsequent to misplacing your thought process.

10. Request help.

I've made it a habit to request help from individuals around me and it's had a stupendous effect in my capacity to get and remain beneficial with whatever the job needing to be done may be for me.

11. Write in a thought book.

Snatch a little scratch pad and scribble down thoughts that come to you for the duration of the day that you would then be able to flip back through in light of the fact that no one can really tell when motivation may strike.

12. Take silent time.

Set aside some time to yourself. Rest with your reflections and simply close your eyes. This isn't simply taking a break, this is tied in with having some isolation in your psyche to watch and tune in to your considerations.

CHAPTER EIGHT

Essential Financial Habits

How well you deal with your funds will direct how much cash you're ready to clutch and even develop over the long time.

1. Track all costs.

Track each and every cost, down to the only remaining penny. Furthermore, do it consistently. Try not to disregard costs. Keep a close eye on them.

2. Open your bills when you got it.

Try not to hold on to open bills. Try not to permit them to accumulate. Open them up, classify and list them so that you're mindful of what should be paid and when.

3. Set aside cash.

You need to save at any rate 20% of your pay each month. At any rate in the event that you truly need to excel.

4. Get up right on time.

Get up early each and every day. A portion of the world's best business people get up at 5 am and prior each and every day.

5. Survey monetary objectives.

Survey your monetary objectives. Do it consistently. Take a legitimate stock of where you remain with your obligation, costs and pay so you can more readily accomplish your cash objectives.

6. Look for monetary motivation.

There are a lot of individuals out there who are able to give you monetary astuteness. Search them out and tune in to their shrewdness and experience so you can carry out it in your own life.

7. Budget constantly.

Learn to budget consistently so you can keep focused. Try not to disregard this. Make a genuine spending plan and stick to it, particularly on the off chance that you experience difficulty dealing with your cash.

8. Put resources into something.

What would you be able to put resources into? Set cash to the side to contribute each day. Regardless of whether it's simply $10.

9. Take a penny minute.

Examine where you remain with a penny minute. Use it to uncover ways you can construct subordinate revenue sources or better adjust your costs.

10. Make shopping records.

Try not to go out on the town to shop without a rundown, else you'll wind up purchasing loads of things that you needn't bother with.

11. Review costs.

Toward the month's end, contrast your receipts with your financial records and bank card consumptions. Does everything add up and synchronize? You'd be astonished on the number of mistakes you may discover when you look.

CHAPTER NINE

<u>Essential health and wellness habits.</u>

At the point when your wellbeing is within proper limits, it's simpler to push forward, develop your business, find an incredible line of work, and accomplish pretty much any objective. The point here is to remain sound, dynamic and fit. Watch what you eat and be careful about anything that goes into your body and understand that poisons like medications and liquor can seriously affect your life.

<u>1. Have breakfast each day.</u>

Breakfast is the main feast of the day. Try not to skip breakfast, regardless of whether it's simply getting something little and brisk.

2. Eat an apple.

An apple every day truly will fend the specialist off. That fiber goes far in your framework to assist with glucose levels, assimilation and that's just the beginning.

3. Rest at any rate 7 hours every evening.

Get plentiful rest every evening. Try not to sleep in, yet additionally don't deny yourself of getting a sound night's rest. It will assist with pressure and uneasiness levels while additionally giving you a decent perspective.

4. Floss and brush your teeth.

Don't simply brush your teeth. Floss. Flossing is significant and assists with battling an assortment of infections.

5. Drink sufficient water.

You need to drink a ton of water for the duration of the day. There are such a large number of advantages to this to disregard it.

6. Eat green vegetables.

Eat green vegetables however much as could be expected. They are a colossal wellspring of alkalinity to assist offset with trip the transcendently acidic eating regimens the vast majority of us have.

7. Walk 10,000 stages per day.

Walk at whatever point you can. Stroll in any event 10,000 stages each day. In case you're feeling fanatical, walk 16,000 stages each day.

8. Eat plentiful fiber.

Fiber is staggeringly significant. Also, getting sufficient measures of fiber through the correct sources ought to be an essential worry of yours.

9. Exercise day by day.

Exercise each and every day, regardless of how short or brief it very well may be for.

CHAPTER TEN

Essential Objective-Oriented Habits

Everybody is focused on accomplishing their objectives, yet not every person is by all accounts ready to arrive. Be that as it may, on the off chance that you track with probably the best habits for accomplishing your objectives, you'll increment your odds of not turning out to be simply one more measurement.

1. Set Brilliant objectives.

Brilliant objectives are significant and will assist you with accomplishing anything. Make certain to set keen objectives consistently.

Meaning of SMART objectives

<u>(S) — Specific (Explicit)</u>

The initial phase in defining a specific objective is to get explicit about it. You should be exact about what the objective is. It can't be left in the theoretical and it should be recorded. Precisely what do you intend to accomplish? A particular objective doesn't simply express that you need to be rich or be a mogul or get more fit. The objective needs to characterize the specific measure of cash you intend to have or the specific measure of weight you plan to lose. Is it 1,000,000 dollars? 10 million dollars? More? Do you intend to shed 20 pounds? 30 pounds? Or on the other hand more perhaps?

Explicit (specific) objectives are undeniably bound to be accomplished. What's more, when they're recorded, you're bound to finish those objectives.

(M) — Meaningful (Significant)

On the off chance that an objective isn't significant, it can't be refined. The identifiable measurement is characterized in the initial step where you get explicit about the objective, however you likewise must have an incredible and sufficient motivation to accomplish it.

Reasons start things out. Answers come next. In the event that you've at any point needed something gravely enough in your life previously, you know exactly how it feels to defeat impediments by making significant objectives. Behind the points of interest of your objective, you must have a sufficient importance. Continue wondering why you need something, at that point attempt to sort out why you need the response to that until the inquiry rises to the appropriate response. A few instances of sufficient reasons would be things like family, opportunity, love, etc.

(A) — Achievable (Reachable)

Set objectives that you can accomplish. Try not to make objectives that are not reachable.

This doesn't imply that you can't set shocking objectives that are farther. You assuredly ought to do that. At the point when you do that, you'll continually search for approaches to accomplish those objectives as long as you make achievements in transit there. Simply ensure that your more limited term objectives are attainable.

Set your destinations on making numerous objectives. Zero in on an entirely feasible year objective, which you can gather speed from. At that point make your 2, 3, 5 and 10-year objectives. This diagram for your life will help provide you guidance with the goal that you realize where you're going. It gives lucidity of direction and determined activities to accomplish the final products. It's an integral asset that dwells in both your cognizant and subliminal personalities when you understand the thing you're pursuing in the long time.

(R) — Relevant (Pertinent)

Your SMART objectives should be applicable to your life. The objectives likewise must be agreeable to your qualities and convictions. What frequently entangles a great many people is that they pick objectives that negate their convictions. Here and there, those objectives even repudiate their guiding principle.

You can't set objectives that are not agreeable with the inward activities of your brain. When circumstances become truly difficult, all things considered, you'll quit on the off chance that you choose to do this.

Pick applicable objectives that are agreeable to your qualities and your convictions and you'll improve over the long time.

(T) — Time Based (Time sensitive)

Brilliant objectives are situated on schedule. They have a careful date that is chosen when those objectives are intended to be accomplished. Assuming you don't choose that date, you're abusing one of the essential destinations of objective setting. At the point when you select a date on a schedule, rather than saying one year from now or the following summer a few years from now, you're bound to finish.

Something else no time like the present based objectives is that you can without much of a stretch make achievements on your way towards that objective. You can separate it into month to month, week after week and surprisingly day by day objectives. It's a lot simpler to zero in on what you need to do today to accomplish an objective, instead of zeroing in on the tremendousness of something that is one year out.

Set aside the effort to choose a particular date on the schedule for your objectives. At that point, put that objective with the date at the top in intense, directly before you on paper on your divider or in your office. Thusly, it's consistently at the forefront of your thoughts and you can allude back to it regularly. You can likewise set it as the foundation screen for your telephone and PC.

2. Objective examination.

Set aside the effort to break down your objectives each and every day. On the off chance that you need to, set day by day objectives or achievements on your approach to accomplishing those greater and more outrageous objectives.

3. Track progress.

Keep tabs on your development towards your objectives consistently. The better you do this, the more probable you'll be to accomplish your objectives after some time.

4. Discover some new information.

What would you be able to adapt today? Regardless of whether you need to simply watch YouTube video to help shed some light regarding a matter, do it.

5. Objective examining.

Go out there and test your objectives. Get pamphlets and begin wanting to make it all the more genuine.

6. Get point of view.

Consider how far you've come. Envision the existences of others. Gain some point of view with the goal that you don't feel disappointed while attempting to accomplish your objectives.

7. Look for direction.

Talk with others who've accomplish large objectives. Ask and look for their direction. You'll be astounded at exactly the number of individuals offer to help you.

CHAPTER ELEVEN

Essential Networking Habits

Networking is a significant piece of progress. Indeed, as the truism goes, your organization is your total assets. How long you burn through networking and how you create and support those connections seriously affects your capacity to prevail at any undertaking.

1. Pose inquiries.

Don't simply discuss yourself. Pose inquiries. Get some answers concerning the other individual. This is imperative to take an interest in the event that you need to prevail with regards to systems administration.

2. Be well presented.

Make certain to prepare yourself day by day. Shower, dress pleasantly and put on your best face and foot forward. No one can really tell what will occur or who you'll meet that can assist with completely changing you.

3. Be straightforward.

Trustworthiness goes far. Try not to attempt to do devious things or guarantee what you can't convey. Continuously under-guarantee and over-convey while organizing.

4. Add esteem.

This is gigantic. Discover ways you can enhance the existences of others. Try not to look for something consequently. Simply add esteem. You'll be astonished at what you get in return.

5. Be positive.

Negative reasoning can consume you for a lifetime.

Be positive. Particularly while organizing with others. You would prefer not to seem to be negative. Make inspiration ongoing in your psyche.

6. Be social.

Approach others. Address them, regardless of whether they don't move toward you. The vast majority are characteristically bashful, and once you move beyond that, the world genuinely is your clam.

7. Offer commendations.

Offering praises is gigantic. Individuals love to be commended so don't limit the force of this habit in networking.

8. Be useful.

Discover ways you can help other people. Pose inquiries and search for cooperative energies where you can assist them with tackling an issue or make up for a shortcoming in their lives.

9. Make presentations.

Continuously make presentations. Do this as regularly as could really be expected. No one can really tell what can emerge from a presentation you make.

10. Sustain contacts.

You need to sustain individuals you come into contact with while organizing. Don't just meet them and disregard them weeks after the fact. Keep in contact as regularly as could really be expected.

CHAPTER TWELVE

<u>Best Profession Habits</u>

Regardless of whether you own your own organization or you work for another person, these are probably the best habits that you can execute in your profession or at the work environment. By remaining steady with these habits, you can guarantee that not exclusively will your endeavors be seen, however you'll remain in front of the famous bend. This takes genuine concentration and responsibility applied reliably over the long run.

<u>1. Show up sooner than expected.</u>

Arrive before you should appear. Continuously. You probably won't receive prompt rewards from this, yet it will go far over the long time.

2. Step up.

Continuously step up. On the off chance that you discover a region for development, follow it. Be proactive and don't trust that individuals will advise you to accomplish something. Do the most measure of work for the most un-beginning return on the off chance that you need to.

3. Put together your workspace.

Go through five minutes every day coordinating your workspace. Regardless of whether it's simply a cabinet or a rack at a time, you'll build force by ordering this habit.

4. Be efficient.

Make rules and frameworks that you can institute and do it consistently. Be efficient about your work to all the more likely arrange and design what you do consistently.

5. Be time-effective.

Try not to sit around idly. Keep in mind, our time is limited. It's restricted. Try not to waste it. Take proprietorship and be dependable to yourself, regardless of whether nobody else is considering you responsible.

6. Take care of an issue.

Become a difficult solver and search for issues that you can address each day. Regardless of whether they're production network related, client related or whatever else, discover them and tackle them head on. Try not to overlook them.

7. Follow up at any rate once.

Be capable and responsible by circling back to individuals consistently. Connect with individuals you didn't hear back from.

8. Be exact.

Exactness is vital in business. Slip-ups are expensive, both from a period viewpoint and a monetary one. Give a valiant effort to twofold and significantly increase check your work consistently.

9. Be snappy.

Try not to sit around or do things more slow than you realize you can do. Obviously, don't forfeit precision for speed, yet assuming you can summon your work faster, do it.

<u>10. Compose clearly.</u>

Practice great composing abilities. From your spelling to your language structure and word utilization, this is significant in business when imparting and reflects back onto the kind of individual you are.

11. Be thorough.

Continuously be intensive and exhaustive in your work. Make a special effort to get things done furthest degree conceivable.

<u>12. Assume liability.</u>

Assume liability for your activities. In the event that you commit errors, own up to them.

13. Be agreeable.

Never markdown the significance of being well disposed with others. Not phony. Not inconsiderate. Simply cordial.

14. Be amenable.

Be benevolent and well mannered. Continuously. Make it a habit. On the off chance that you see yourself veering away from this, upset the example, apologize and execute this habit whatever it takes.

CHAPTER THIRTEEN

Essential Structural Habits

Getting coordinated and remaining coordinated is vital for your prosperity. Indeed, examines have recommended that actual mess can degrade us from accomplishing our objectives. That may be the reason they say, clean house, clean psyche. So work to clean up your home and office, since it will assist you with accomplishing your fundamental objectives.

1. Give everything a home.

Invest a touch of energy consistently giving things a home, where you can return them after they've been utilized.

2. Coordinate in segments.

Start with a cabinet here and a rack there and systematically go through until everything is coordinated, even your PC's work area and organizers.

3. Perfect as you go.

Clean in areas. Do one little space each day in case you're experiencing difficulty with this. After you utilize the shower, clean it once each week, or the latrine or the kitchen, or elsewhere so far as that is concerned.

4. Utilize a schedule.

Execute a schedule framework that you can establish to remain coordinated with your day and keep you on target.

5. Make records.

Continuously make records for all that requires to be finished. Track things and cross them off in each part of your life (not simply to-do things).

6. Try not to stall.

Keep the 15-minute guideline. Set a clock on your cell phone for 15 minutes. Tackle whatever you have been putting away for a long time in 15 minutes; do not put it off again.

7. Excuse your internal pundit.

We as a whole have a negative voice in our psyches. Yet, the better you are at excusing your inward pundit, the more advancement you'll make in an assortment of parts of your life.

8. Be definitive.

Settle on brisk choices and change them gradually.

Be conclusive of what you need and seek after with

a determined energy.

9. Survey and focus on.

Continuously survey and focus on the things that

should be finished. Sort out how significant they are

on the great plan of things and put the perfect

measure of exertion towards them.

www.ingramcontent.com/pod-product-compliance
Lightning Source LLC
Chambersburg PA
CBHW050039260726

48658CB00005B/1683